DR. DAVID EIFRIG JR., MD, MBA
with the Stansberry Research team

THE LIVING
CURE

THE PROMISE OF CANCER
IMMUNOTHERAPY

Published by Stansberry Research

Edited by Carli Flippen and Fawn Gwynallen

About Stansberry Research

Founded in 1999 and based out of Baltimore, Maryland, Stansberry Research is the largest independent source of financial insight in the world. It delivers unbiased investment advice to self-directed investors seeking an edge in a wide variety of sectors and market conditions.

Stansberry Research has nearly two dozen analysts and researchers – including former hedge-fund managers and buy-side financial experts. They produce a steady stream of timely research on value investing, income generation, resources, biotech, financials, short-selling, macroeconomic analysis, options trading, and more.

The company's unrelenting and uncompromised insight has made it one of the most respected and sought-after research organizations in the financial sector. It has nearly one million readers and more than 500,000 paid subscribers in over 100 countries.

About the Author

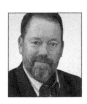 Dr. Eifrig is the editor of three Stansberry Research newsletters... His largest monthly publication, *Retirement Millionaire,* shows 100,000-plus readers how to live a millionaire lifestyle on less money than you'd imagine possible. *Retirement Trader* shows readers a safe way to double or triple the gains in their retirement accounts with less risk. *Income Intelligence* shows investors how to analyze the income markets to maximize their income and total returns.

Doc has one of the best track records in the financial-newsletter business. From 2010 to 2014, he closed 136 winning positions in a row for his *Retirement Trader* subscribers.

Before joining Stansberry Research in 2008, Dr. Eifrig worked in arbitrage and trading groups with major Wall Street investment banks, including Goldman Sachs, Chase Manhattan, and Yamaichi in Japan. He has also published peer-reviewed medical research. After retiring from Wall Street, Dr. Eifrig attended medical school to become a board-eligible ophthalmologist. At Stansberry Research, he shares his love for empowering people with his finance and medical knowledge.

Table of Contents

Introduction

Nearly 1.7 million Americans every year get a diagnosis that would chill any of us...

"You have cancer."

A physician friend of mine delivers this three-word phrase over and over to patients every week.

When talking with her, you can almost feel her pain and the emotional toll it takes. When she's "on-call covering the service" for a week at a time, she has to schedule a massage at the end of the week just to physically recharge herself.

And of course, that's nothing compared with the trauma newly diagnosed patients suffer. Hearing the news you have cancer can devastate people. It changes your whole world.

Cancer kills one in four Americans, making it the second-most common cause of death after heart disease. That's nearly half-a-million Americans dying from cancer each year. More than 1.5 million new cases are diagnosed annually.

You can also gauge cancer's toll in the dollars spent to fight it... In 2013, the U.S. government funded $4.8 billion in cancer research. The average health care spending on a cancer patient is around $20,000 annually for treatment (with patients paying less than one-tenth that).

All told, more than $125 billion is spent on cancer care per year, just in the United States.

Virtually everyone has at some point watched a spouse, family member, or a close friend struggle with the disease. And if you haven't, you will.

Sadly, despite all the money and effort we've spent to battle cancer over the years, we've made little progress in overcoming cancer's lethal power.

The death rates for cancers like breast, prostate, colorectal, liver, and pancreatic haven't changed significantly since the 1930s. By comparison, stroke and heart disease death rates fell 74% and 64%, respectively, between 1950 and 2006.

That's in large part because the basic weapons in our arsenal to fight cancer – surgery, chemotherapy, and radiation – haven't changed in decades.

Until now...

I've written this booklet to introduce as many people as possible to what I believe is the most significant breakthrough in fighting cancer since the development of chemotherapy in the 1940s... and perhaps ever.

An emerging class of cancer treatments is proving itself to be more powerful at battling the disease than anything developed in the past 120 years. Thanks to these treatments, patients with some of the *deadliest cancers* are being declared cancer-free.

The advances I want to tell you about today are 100% based in science... tested by doctors and biologists in peer-reviewed studies at the world's leading cancer research centers.

I'm not talking about any new surgical techniques, advanced forms of radiation treatment, or potent new chemotherapy drugs.

Instead, these treatments unleash a *living cure* that is coded into the human body...

Although the most recent advances in cancer treatment haven't gotten the kind of mainstream media coverage they deserve, the research and results of these new treatments make one thing clear...

The power to defeat cancer is already inside our bodies.

The trick is unleashing our immune system's army on the disease...

This realization is changing everything about how we approach cancer.

This booklet includes a listing of the published studies and related research we relied on in this report... so you can read the science yourself and show it to your doctor. (You can find it in the "Further Reading" section at the end of the booklet.)

More important, I'm going to show you...

- Why your own immune system is probably the most powerful tool against cancer.

- How to access clinical trials, and where some of the most promising work is being done.

- What questions you absolutely must ask your doctor... and any future members of your medical team... *immediately* after a cancer diagnosis.

I've also included a second section to this booklet that details critical information anyone who has been diagnosed with cancer needs to know... whether or not you choose to take advantage of the "Living Cure."

This information is so important, I'm giving it away for free. And I encourage you to share it with anyone who has been diagnosed with cancer... or has a loved one facing the disease.

But before we delve into the science, I want to show you how powerful the "Living Cure" can be...

— Part I —

The Secret Weapon Inside You

Chapter 1

The Quiet Revolution

In 2012, six-year-old Emily Whitehead was facing the end of a two-year battle with acute lymphoblastic leukemia, a cancer of the blood.

It was a battle she was losing. Emily had relapsed twice after chemotherapy. Doctors said her organs would fail within days. In desperation, her family agreed to try the experimental Living Cure treatment...

Three weeks after receiving this treatment at the Children's Hospital of Philadelphia, she was found to be in complete remission. She is still cancer-free more than two years later.

Arrica Wallace, a 34-year-old mother of two, was given less than a year to live after her metastatic Stage 3 cervical cancer spread to the lymph nodes in her abdomen and chest.

She received a form of the Living Cure treatment through a National Institutes of Health clinical trial. Four months later, all the tumors had disappeared. She has shown no signs of recurrence for nearly two years.

And Mary Elizabeth Williams, also a mother of two and a writer for the website Salon.com, had Stage 4 melanoma – one of the deadliest known cancers. It had spread to her lungs and back. The average life span for people with Williams' diagnosis is less than a year.

Williams received a combination of two experimental drugs – among the first of their kind – through Memorial Sloan Kettering Cancer Center in New York. She was cancer-free within three months... and still is.

I read a dozen medical journals on a regular basis. I attend at least four national medical conferences every year. Many of my friends and family members work at some of the top cancer centers in the world. Stories like the ones above border on miraculous. But we are seeing more and more of them... It's clear we're on the cusp of a revolution in cancer therapy.

But it's a quiet revolution. The public is largely shut out of the world of scientific research. Advances in the lab take *years* to reach ordinary folks. And many general practice doctors (even some specialists) don't keep up with the latest research.

That's why I've put together this booklet. To introduce you to the lifesaving revolution called **immunotherapy**.

At its heart, immunotherapy is a simple concept. Our bodies attack foreign invaders – germs, bacteria, viruses – with a powerful army of natural defenses. What if we could turn our immune system on cancerous cells?

The concept of using the body's army to battle cancer goes back more than 120 years to a physician named Dr. William Coley...

In 1891, William Coley was on a mission. He had spent weeks scouring New York's Lower East Side, looking for one man.

A respected doctor and surgeon, Coley had been reduced to one job: Find Fred Stein.

Stein was a German immigrant in his late 30s who worked as a housepainter. He was a fairly normal guy, except in one respect...

Eleven years earlier, Stein was suffering from a fast-growing tumor in his neck. Despite four surgeries to remove it, doctors had deemed Stein's case "absolutely hopeless." He was destined to die from it.

But then, Stein contracted a bacterial infection on his face. Without the benefit of antibiotics, he had to let his body fight it off.

Miraculously... Stein didn't just beat the infection... *he beat the cancer.* Something about the way his immune system strengthened to fight the bacteria led his body to attack and defeat the cancer. Stein made a full recovery.

When Coley read about Stein's case, he knew he had to find him. He might hold the key to finding a cure for cancer.

You see, Coley had spent years researching a controversial idea...

He believed that the body's own immune system was a far more powerful weapon against cancer than anyone imagined... Coley thought that an immune response against cancer could be "awakened" by making people sick with other kinds of infections.

For Stein, the infected wound on his face did the trick.

Coley developed a vaccine based on the bacteria that had infected Stein. He later created two other harmful bacteria that were "deactivated" (in other words, killed) prior to injection.

If this sounds a little crazy, keep in mind, this is still how vaccines work today.

We help our bodies develop immunity to deadly viruses and bacteria by giving them a "taste" of the pathogen.

Sometimes, it's a deactivated version. And sometimes, it's what's called a "live attenuated" version – a live strain that has been weakened so you don't get the disease.

Measles, mumps, tetanus, polio – you name it: That's how we've defeated many of the world's deadliest diseases.

The science that has brought us these immunizations is an absolute marvel of human progress. But in the end, it's still our own immune systems doing all the work. Coley understood this.

Whether it's a real sickness or a vaccine that mimics the real thing... these threats awaken a powerful immune response from the body.

That's why people sometimes feel side effects and a bit "under the weather" for a few days after getting a vaccine. Those symptoms are the telltale signs of your immune system going into overdrive.

And that's what Coley was trying to harness with his vaccine. It was a primitive form of immunotherapy, and he used it to treat hundreds of patients over the years.

He was not always successful. Some patients had terrible side effects.

Some did not survive. But many patients' tumors shrank and disappeared completely – just like Stein's – and lived normal lives for years before dying of unrelated causes.

In fact, Coley demonstrated that even the so-called "side effects" – particularly fever – have powerful healing functions. Even in modern day, pediatricians recommend allowing fevers (as long as they are below 105 degrees) to run their course in many cases.

Unfortunately, Coley's results weren't as consistent as the competing approach at the time – radiation. In the ensuing battle to beat the disease, radiation won out as the preferred treatment for more than a century.

Coley was overshadowed by a rival doctor, James Ewing, who also happened to be Coley's boss. Ewing was an early advocate of radiation therapy and actually forbid Coley from using his treatment on patients, despite its success.

But the idea of immunotherapy was pushed aside for another reason, too...

As we started to learn more about cancer in the early 20th century, researchers realized that it is very different from infectious diseases like measles or the flu.

Cancer originates inside the body, due mostly (we now know) to damage to our DNA that causes cell growth to run amok.

Unfortunately, the medical community drew the wrong conclusion from that insight. They figured... if it isn't an infectious disease, it can't be healed by the immune system.

Today, we know that Coley was on to something...

Cancer is an extremely complex disease. Since Coley's time, we've learned volumes about things like how it starts, the ways it grows, the differences between the varieties, and how cancerous cells function.

Without that information, Coley couldn't figure out why the immune system beat a few cancers, but not others. If he could have applied today's knowledge, he may have convinced others to work on his idea of using the immune system to beat cancer.

Because now, it appears to work.

Cancer has a lot of moving parts and a lot of causes. Over time, the research focus has shifted from attacking one or another of these aspects. At times, the "hot" research has focused on chemotherapy mega-dosing, the viral foundations of some cancer strains, the genomic aspects of specific tumors, and others.

Immunotherapy has a long history of stepping in and out of the spotlight for cancer research. The 2014 presentations at the American Society of Clinical Oncology (ASCO) – a major national cancer-research conference – were concentrated on these new treatments. So it's worth looking into how they developed from Coley's original work.

What Is Cancer?

There are more than 100 types of cancer, but these can be categorized into five main groups.

Carcinomas are the main type of cancer and the most often diagnosed. These are cancers of your "organs" – like your lungs, pancreas, colon, bladder, breasts, even skin.

Sarcomas are much less common and form either in the bone or in soft tissues like nerves, blood vessels, cartilage, or muscle.

Lymphomas are cancers of the cells in the lymph system, the network in your body that moves excess blood plasma and immune cells throughout the body.

Leukemias are cancers of the blood cells, like white blood cells.

And the last, **melanomas**, are cancers of the pigment cells in your skin (not to be confused with carcinomas of the skin).

— Chapter 2 —

History of Immunotherapy

The idea of using infections to stimulate the immune system to fight cancer can be traced back through medical history all the way to the ancient Egyptians.

In some Egyptian records from around 1550 BC, the renowned physician Imhotep had prescribed wrapping tumors (or just swellings) with moist salves made of plants and minerals coupled with an open incision. This type of treatment easily induces infections to the site, suggesting that the introduction of an infection could be the earliest form of treating cancers.

Other cases in history reported tumors disappearing after a patient encountered an infection – sometimes unrelated to the tumor.

Doctors in the 1700s and 1800s expanded the idea of infections stimulating the immune system to fight cancer. Prescriptions at the time included wrapping affected areas in septic bandages or introducing infections like erysipelas or syphilis.

Around the same time Coley suggested using infections to help the body's immune system "kick on" and fight cancer, Dr. Joseph Lister's sterilization procedures for surgery became accepted as standards of practice. In a business where germs were now the enemy, the idea of introducing more germs seemed ludicrous.

The medical community went so far as to criticize a published discussion on using infections to fight cancer by saying the idea would "make surgery go backwards." Germs were now understood to cause disease and had to be avoided.

By the 1930s, radiation therapy was becoming a standard treatment for cancer in addition to surgery. Since radiation suppresses the immune system, immune-based therapies seemed counterproductive.

The big breakthrough came in the 1960s and 1970s through the research of Dr. Lloyd Old at the Memorial Sloan Kettering Cancer Center in New York. Old discovered that although tumor cells have the same chemical signatures as healthy cells, they do have unique types of surface proteins. These proteins could be targeted by the immune system if they could be identified.

Not long afterward, Dr. James Allison of the University of California, Berkeley started his research into specific switches to turn the immune system "on." (More on this in a moment).

Allison is probably the person most responsible for the lifesaving advances available today. If cancer is ever cured for good... he may be the one the world has to thank.

Allison lost his mother to lymphoma, his uncles to melanoma and lung cancer, and his brother to prostate cancer. He also had prostate cancer himself... although he was successfully treated by having his prostate removed in 2005.

So researching cancer was personal for him. And Allison knew he wanted to focus on the immune system.

That was no easy decision. Allison was moving up through the academic ranks at a time when immunotherapy was still considered quackery. "It had such a bad rap," Allison told a reporter. "People would say to me, 'Don't do tumor immunology, it'll ruin your reputation.'"

But Texas-born Allison had always had a rebellious streak. He had refused to take a high school science course that didn't teach evolution. He graduated at 16.

For a while, he preferred playing the harmonica to researching tumors. He even convinced Willie Nelson to come to an open-mic where he sometimes played... and ended up sharing the stage with him.

As his research developed, he used to go to conferences to share his results – only to find his lecture rooms empty. Immunotherapy wasn't a big draw. People weren't interested.

Some nonspecific immunotherapy drugs, like interferon, had failed to produce good results. So drug companies had lost interest in pursuing additional immunotherapies against cancer. That field of research was considered dead.

Still, a few researchers, like Allison, persisted. And in 1990, the Food and Drug Administration (FDA) approved the first immunotherapy drug – a vaccine initially made to protect against tuberculosis. The vaccine, called BCG, is made from live attenuated (weakened) bacteria called mycobacterium bovis, the bacteria that leads to tuberculosis in cattle.

Used to treat bladder cancer, BCG is injected directly into the bladder. The bacteria find their way into immune cells called "macrophages" that trigger the full immune system response. The bacteria also enter the cancer cells and wind up marking them for elimination, too, thus knocking out the tumor. Even decades later, BCG is still the best treatment available for bladder cancer.

Allison collaborated with drug company Medarex to produce ipilimumab. After a long process,

How Cancer Grows

Cancer grows in two ways. First, it grows on itself. Imagine a tumor just growing from the size of a pea to the size of a golf ball, for example. Cancer can also grow outward. By moving to other organs or tissues, cancer cells can spread throughout the body and continue growing in places far different from where they began. This is known as "metastasis."

Your doctor will determine how far your cancer has progressed at the time of your diagnosis. This is often done by stages. In general terms, cancer stages go like this:

Stage 0 – Cancer is in original place and has not spread.

Stage 1, 2, and 3 – Tumor has grown and/or spread to nearby locations. The higher the stage number, the further the growth.

Stage 4 – The cancer has metastasized, or spread to distant areas of the body.

Staging also takes into account whether the cancer has spread to the lymph nodes. Cancer that invades lymph nodes can travel more easily to other parts of the body.

ipilimumab received approval from the FDA in 2011 to treat patients in the late stages of the skin cancer melanoma.

Ipilimumab has amazing effects on melanoma patients. More than 20% of the patients receiving the drug end up surviving long term... a vast improvement for the kind of cancer it treats. In some patients, the cancer completely disappears.

Ipilimumab has now been studied in 2,901 patients in more than 25 clinical trials. Responses to it have been not only favorable, but have prolonged survival in advanced Stage 4 melanoma – a truly remarkable feat.

Immunotherapy has already helped patients with melanoma, prostate, and bladder cancer. It has shown positive results in experimental studies for kidney, pancreatic, and some lung cancer. Different forms of immunotherapy "reprogram" the patient's own immune system cells. Other forms create artificial chemical tags that mark cancer cells for destruction.

How do these therapies work? To understand immunotherapy, we first need to understand our own immune system.

Chapter 3

How Your Body Marshals Its Army Against Cancer

The body's immune system consists of many different cell types. Cells like macrophages generally destroy invading cells by engulfing them and breaking them down. They work in response to cells like "B" and "T" cells.

B and T cells trigger what's called "antigen-dependent stimulation" of immune responses. That might sound like a mouthful. But it simply means these cells latch onto enemy cells and break them down either on their own or by signaling for back up. Their response depends on the "antigen" or the specific chemical tag on an enemy cell.

In addition, your plasma cells produce antibodies, proteins that attach to specific receptors on enemy cells. When a pathogen enters your body, many parts of your immune system rally to fight it off. These antibodies are the last line of defense. These Y-shaped proteins have a section in the top fork that matches specific proteins. This fork will attach to those proteins on the outside of an enemy cell.

Antibodies work in one of three ways. First, when they bind to the enemy cell's protein, they can clog up the proteins and prohibit the cell from carrying out activities or trigger a chemical response within the cell that will shut it down. Second, they can trigger other immune cells to come and kill the enemy cell. Third, they can create inflammation, which makes it much harder for the enemy cell to move around. Keeping enemy cells localized makes them easier to kill.

Take a look at the graphic on the next page. It breaks down the "antigen-dependent stimulation" of immune responses...

BASIC ANTIBODY PATHWAY

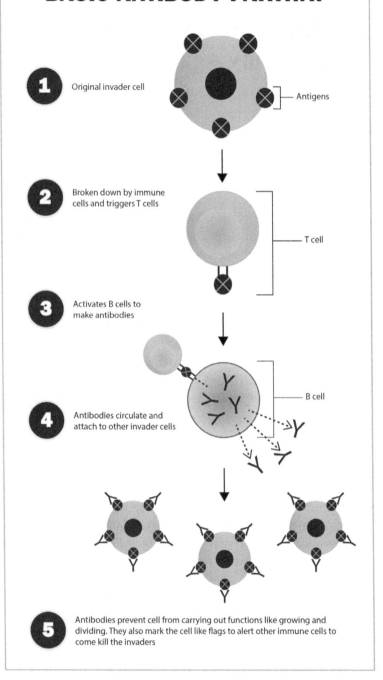

1 Original invader cell

Antigens

2 Broken down by immune cells and triggers T cells

T cell

3 Activates B cells to make antibodies

B cell

4 Antibodies circulate and attach to other invader cells

5 Antibodies prevent cell from carrying out functions like growing and dividing. They also mark the cell like flags to alert other immune cells to come kill the invaders

— Chapter 4 —

How Immunotherapy Works

Immunotherapy aims to stimulate different parts of the immune system to effectively get your body to fight its own cells – cancer cells.

There are three main types of cancer-targeted immunotherapy. The first kind is called nonspecific immunotherapy. Drugs in this class activate your immune system as a whole instead of targeting the attack. These include the interleukin and interferon drugs, which have had mixed results.

The second type is the kind Allison researched. It uses something called monoclonal antibodies (or mAbs for short). Antibodies, just like those your body produces in response to the flu vaccine, can be made in a lab and specifically tailored to fight almost any kind of protein marker.

The man-made antibodies have special chemical coding in the Y branch of their fork-like structure. This allows them to find and latch onto the special proteins on cancer cells. This either shuts down the cell through a chemical chain reaction or signals your other immune cells to come and kill those cells.

Antibody-focused immunotherapy is at the forefront of cancer research today. It strives to solve one of the biggest problems with cancer treatment: Cancer cells are not foreign bodies, like bacteria, that drugs can easily target. Since our own bodies' cells make them, they can easily "camouflage" themselves. The cancerous cells have no chemical thumbprint that signals them as "different" or "dangerous." So immune cells pass by the cancer cells and read them as normal.

How can your immune cells track down a cell that has the same chemical "thumbprint" as the body's healthy cells?

That's what drove Dr. Allison's research. In 1978, Allison started trying to get a specific type of white blood cell, T cells, to attack tumors.

It turns out that T cells are like high-performance racecars. Their capabilities are astounding... but only if you turn on the ignition, step on the gas pedal... and release the brakes.

Before Allison, researchers didn't even know that these switches existed.

Allison found all three.

The first switch was an antigen receptor that the T cell uses to "read" the surface antigens of tumor cells. This was the ignition switch needed to make T cells go.

The second switch was a T-cell surface molecule called CD28. Scientists call it a "co-stimulatory" receptor.

In other words, even if the ignition is on... if you don't activate CD28, the T cell doesn't go. It was the gas pedal.

But Allison's third discovery was the one that changed immunotherapy forever.

In the fall of 2005, Allison was studying another T-cell surface marker called cytotoxic T-lymphocyte antigen-4, or CTLA-4.

This molecule is responsible for "putting the brakes on" the T cell's killing spree. It prevents T cells from running rampant and killing the body's own cells. When self-antigens (like those on cancer cells and healthy cells) are present, CTLA-4 switches off the T cell.

Allison figured out how to switch it back on.

To get T cells to fight cancer cells, Allison focused on CTLA-4. He found that blocking this protein caused the T cells to attack tumors.

By implementing the same method that other researchers use to create man-made antibodies, Allison created an antibody targeted to shut off CTLA-4. His drug, ipilimumab, is the first of its kind.

CTLA-4 isn't the only pathway that cancer uses to shut down immune response. Various studies have identified another, even more important, receptor on the surface of activated T cells known as PD-1. This is a programmed cell death receptor. It's designed to be activated by healthy cells to make sure that the immune system doesn't harm healthy tissue.

For example, fetus cells are covered with PD-1. It's nature's way of making sure mom's immune system doesn't attack the "foreign" baby cells.

Cancerous cells make lots of PD-1 signaling proteins so that they can turn off any killer T cells that show up. Cancer essentially uses PD-1 to disguise itself as fetal cells and keep the immune system at bay.

What's important about PD-1 research is that PD-1 is also a receptor on B cells. By using antibodies to shut off PD-1, both your T cells and B cells can launch a stronger, more widespread attack on cancer cells.

The biggest news out of ASCO in 2014 was a large clinical trial using a newly developed PD-1 signal-blocking antibody (MK-3475) by Merck in combination with ipilimumab (Yervoy). This was the largest Phase I study ever in oncology. Dr. Antoni Ribas at UCLA conducted the trial with more than 400 patients, most of whom had cancers that had failed to fully respond to Yervoy alone.

This combination study produced staggering results – almost unbelievable to the oncology community. Patients with late-stage melanoma have an average life span of nine months. Those who fail treatment with Yervoy are usually just days or weeks away from dying. But the one-year survival rate in this study was 85% and the two-year survival rate was 79%.

There has never been anything like these survival rates in late-stage cancer therapy. Using Merck's PD-1 antibody and Yervoy, Ribas reduced tumor size in 72% of the patients. Only 8% of the patients experienced side effects.

Commenting on the results from this study, Dr. Ryan Sullivan, professor at Harvard Medical School, said of the MK-3475 antibody: "I think that this drug is the best new anticancer drug that is available today."

The FDA fast-tracked approval of this new drug in September 2014. Not only did it gain approval, but Merck's new drug carries the specific recommendation to be used in conjunction with ipilimumab. Promising new combination therapies are everywhere in today's oncology research.

The third type of immunotherapy is cancer vaccines. These vaccines include both preventive vaccines (like the one for human papilloma virus, or HPV) and a few cancer-fighting vaccines (such as Sipuleucel-T, which is used to treat prostate cancer). Preventive vaccines focus on stopping certain viruses known to cause cancer, like HPV, HIV, and Hepatitis B & C.

Cancer-fighting vaccines are still in the early stages of development. In principle, they work by taking the patient's immune cells (usually T cells) out of their body, exposing them to chemicals or to a modified virus, then injecting the "reprogrammed" T cells back into the patient. The new T cells have been programmed to find and destroy specific proteins on cancer cells. This is different from BCG, which can be made in batches, because it requires each patient's own cells.

The only approved cancer-fighting vaccine right now is Sipuleucel-T. To make this vaccine, a patient's own immune cells are collected then exposed to chemicals that induce the cells to respond to a prostate-cancer-specific protein called PAP. The modified cells are injected back into the patient. Those cells then begin an immune response to PAP. This process, called adoptive T-cell transfer, is being studied in new trials right now for cancers like leukemia.

In a 2012 trial in Philadelphia, 12 patients with advanced leukemia received this type of treatment, which helped their T cells seek out and kill B cells that had turned cancerous. In the trial, three adults had complete remissions, four improved but did not have full remissions, and one was not evaluated at the time the results were reported. Two adults did not have any response. Two children were also treated – one relapsed, but the other had a full remission. The results, although mixed, have provided hope for remission for a devastating advanced-stage disease.

One of the common misperceptions is that immunotherapy is a "natural" cure for cancer without any of the side effects you have with chemotherapy or radiation.

On the contrary, the high stimulation of T cells can make them run rampant on other body systems, too. So not only can they attack the cancer cells, but they can attack the skin, intestines, liver, thyroid, and other organs. There have been reports of severe intestinal inflammation that could lead to death if not treated immediately.

The main issues with immunotherapy have to do with the complex nature of cancer. As we described, antibody-driven therapies target specific tags on cancer cells. But even when a patients has the cancer targeted by the drug, his or her individual form of cancer may not have the needed "tag" that allows the therapy to work.

To make it even more complex, some cancer cells can have high mutation rates – meaning it can be only a matter of time before the tag that the therapy targets can "disappear" in the new cancer cells, allowing the cancer to survive.

Although some immunotherapies have shown tremendous potential and promising results, one of the major limitations is that they have been treated as a "last-ditch" effort. In many trials, the drugs are only given at the most advanced stage. Late stages of cancer also weaken the immune system, meaning a full response to treatment may not occur.

Is Immunotherapy About to Go Mainstream?

Immunotherapy is starting to join the trifecta of standard care for cancer – surgery, radiation, and chemotherapy. As cancer researcher Dr. Steven Rosenberg said in an interview with Frontline Medicine, "We desperately need new approaches to treatment, and immunotherapy is now joining the mainstream. And in some cases, is going to replace chemotherapy as a systemic treatment."

Surgery and radiation are not "systemic." They only attack what the surgeon or the radiation beam focuses on. Since cancer cells spread to other parts of the body, only chemotherapy so far has been able to go after those wayward cells and kill them. Immunotherapy is now joining that fight by using the immune system to track down and kill cancer cells wherever they may be.

Presentations at the 2014 Immunotherapies and Vaccine Summit showed promising trials combining therapies as well. Dr. James Welsh from the MD Anderson Cancer Center detailed how the combination of localized radiation therapy can actually help stimulate systemic immune response when used with immunotherapy treatments.

Other presenters focused on how combining different types of immunotherapies can enhance their effects.

For example, using anti-PD-1 therapy in some cancers may induce only a partial immune response. Combining it with other drivers like monoclonal antibodies could give it enough of a boost to push a full-blown systemic response.

But just as chemotherapy has side effects, so does immunotherapy. Shutting down immune system inhibitors can open the door for your immune cells to attack normal tissue. In ipilimumab, for example, about 15% of patients developed severe colitis. In other words, their immune systems attacked the lining of their colon, leading to severe – sometimes deadly – diarrhea. In anti-PD-1 drugs, too, the immune system has been seen to attack healthy lung tissue in some patients.

I'm not against chemotherapy... even though it has serious drawbacks and its effectiveness has been exaggerated by bad medicine. In fact, it turns out that *chemotherapy and immunotherapy can be a powerful combo-punch.*

When chemotherapy drugs attack cancer cells, they burst those cells open – releasing a flood of the tumor-specific antigens that stimulate the immune system. Immunotherapy can then use those antigens to stimulate the immune system to wage war on the cancer cells.

— Chapter 5 —

The Promise of the Living Cure

In 2002, doctors diagnosed Doug Olson with chronic lymphocytic leukemia... a cancer that begins in the patient's bone marrow.

Chronic lymphocytic leukemia is a slow-to-develop but hard-to-cure form of blood cancer.

Olson began his fight. But after eight years and four failed attempts to beat his cancer through traditional treatments, his condition was worsening. That's when he joined a clinical trial testing a new way...

In the summer of 2010, Olson became the third person to receive genetically modified T cells. As part of the trial, Dr. Carl June of the Penn Abramson Cancer Center would gather T cells from the patient. The researchers would then reprogram them so that when reintroduced into the patient's body, the T cells would hunt down and kill the cancer cells.

At first, the treatment made Olson miserable... The reintroduction triggered something called a "cytokine storm" – an overload of T cell response, which caused him to develop a raging fever and flu-like symptoms that put him in the hospital.

But a week later, Olson emerged without a trace of cancer in his body. "Pounds of tumor went away in a week," June said in a video statement released by Penn Medicine.

Three years later, Olson is still in remission. Even better, *there's promise that these reprogrammed T cells will protect Olson in the future*, continuing to survive and guard against any relapse. June says this team not only can't find any cancer cells in Olson's body, but they can still see some of the reprogrammed T cells still living and active in his body.

This is an incredible achievement for a chronic condition...

But still, there's an immense amount we need to learn about how to train our bodies' armies against cancer cells.

For example... as we described in Doug Olson's story, the promise behind the Living Cure of immunotherapy is that the immune system will learn the mutated proteins on a cancer cell, recognize them as foreign, and remember to fight them in the future.

You have special T cells called memory T cells that aid in this process. It's the same way we develop immunity through vaccines today. Your body recognizes the dead or the attenuated portions of a known disease from a vaccine and builds antibody resistance. Your T cells learn to fight this type of invader.

So if the immune system fights cancer cells, shouldn't the body remember to fight those same cells in the future?

The answer isn't very simple. There are durability studies out there suggesting that people like Olson will retain memory T cells that will continue to fight similar cancer cells in the future. However, this research is still new and developing. Long-term survival and continued remission have yet to be proven.

To make matters more complicated, modified T cells or monoclonal antibodies only fight one specific type of cancer. If you initially receive immunotherapy for melanoma, will it also fight off the pancreatic cancer you develop 10 years later?

The answer is: We're not sure yet.

You see, while stories like Olson's are extremely promising, not all cancers respond the same way to immunotherapy. Dr. Steven Rosenberg, chief of the Surgery Branch at the National Cancer Institute, expressed the main concern with immunotherapy treatments...

> The immune system is so exquisitely sensitive and specific that even tiny amounts of a molecule on the cancer that's present also on normal tissues can result in the destruction of the cancer, but the normal tissues as well. So it's this search for targets expressed by the cancer and not the normal tissue that represents a major obstacle to progress.

Every cancer has different mutations. These mutations are what cause them to grow without stopping, replicate much more rapidly, and spread to other parts of the body. Melanoma, for example, has more than the usual amount of genetic mutations. This results in more mutated proteins on the cell's surface. More mutated proteins means the immune system has an easier time recognizing these cells as "foreign."

It's this simple fact that makes melanoma a prime target for immunotherapy. Since the immune system already recognizes the melanoma cells as foreign, it has an easier time being programmed to kill them. The same is true with lung cancer caused by smoking – more mutations in this type of cancer lead to easier recognition of the cancer cells as foreign invaders that need to be destroyed.

That makes cancers like leukemia, melanoma, and lung cancer all beneficiaries of immunotherapy. On the other hand, epithelial cancers, like those of the breast, prostate, ovary, and esophagus, have fewer mutations and are easily passed over by the immune system. Fewer mutations also make immunotherapy much more difficult since the body views these cancer cells as "self" and will not destroy them as easily. These types of cancers account for 90% of cancer deaths in the U.S. So finding those "targets" specific to each cancer type is crucial for the progression of immunotherapy research.

And that's exactly where researchers like Rosenberg are focusing their new trials. New studies are being conducted every day on different types of cancers, and the search to pinpoint those targets continues. For example, in his interview, he discussed his lab is now beginning one of the first studies on how to target immunotherapy on breast cancer.

The final problem ties into these mutations as well. Cancer can mutate and every person's cancer is just a bit different because of their individual genetic makeup. That's why the future of immunotherapy lies in using genetic research to further personalize – and therefore better target – cancer treatments.

Rosenberg is optimistic about the future. "Now there's a lot of opportunity on the horizon as we marry modern genomic science with modern immunotherapy to develop treatments that will be highly specific to the cancer." The next wave of cancer medicine is here and will only get better as we further tailor our treatments to individual cancer mutations.

Science magazine named cancer immunotherapy the breakthrough of the year for 2013... on par with past breakthroughs such as sequencing the entire human genome and cloning a living mammal.

Allison also won the 2014 Breakthrough Prize in Life Sciences, a $3 million award. And the head of the MD Anderson Cancer Center, where Allison works, thinks Allison will eventually win the Nobel Prize as well. We are standing on the edge of the new frontier of cancer treatment.

— Chapter 6 —

Where You Can Find the Best Cancer Treatment

No matter what type of cancer you have, finding the best place to undergo any treatment – whether standard chemotherapy and radiation or a cutting-edge immunotherapy trial – is essential to your success fighting cancer.

Hospitals across the U.S. specialize in the research and treatment of certain cancers, and it's critical you find them if you want to survive.

While the doctor who diagnosed you may have some suggestions, it's important to do your own research. Treatments are constantly evolving, so your doctor may not have all of the latest information.

A good place to start is the National Cancer Institute (NCI).

NCI was founded in 1937 and makes up one part of the National Institutes of Health (NIH). The NCI is responsible for conducting cutting-edge cancer research, providing funding for other research projects, and educating doctors and the public about cancer diagnosis and treatments.

The NCI has 68 "Designated Cancer Centers" in the U.S. These

For Readers Outside the U.S.

While we're focusing on cancer in the U.S., organizations around the world are dedicated to helping cancer patients and working toward cures.

If you're in the United Kingdom, Cancer Research UK offers information on doctors who specialize in certain cancers, clinical trials, and how to find support groups and counseling. And it's entirely publicly funded.

You can find similar foundations in other countries across the globe. Ask your doctor if he's familiar with any or simply look up cancer research in your country on an online search engine.

state-of-the-art centers are often leaders in advancements in cancer detection and treatment. You can find the list of NCI-designated cancer centers here: http://cancercenters.cancer.gov/center/cancercenters.

The NCI also has 64 highly specialized treatment and clinical trial centers that focus on specific types of cancer – called Specialized Programs of Research Excellence (SPOREs) – spread across 20 states.

The list is divided into "organ" locations. For example, if you're looking for SPOREs for liver cancer, you'd look under "Gastrointestinal" in the organ-location list.

Below, we've listed the top five deadliest cancers, based on their average five-year survival rates.

Top Five Deadliest Cancers	
Cancer	Five-Year Survival Rates*
Pancreas	6%
Liver	15%
Lung and Bronchus	16%
Esophagus	17%
Stomach	27%
Source: American Cancer Society	*Average across all stages

If you or someone you know has one of these five cancers, we encourage you to go to the closest SPORE for your treatment. These centers often have the best doctors and treatments for specific cancers. So while some of these may be far from you, if getting the best care gives you a better chance at living, consider the expenses you might incur.

Take a look at this map of the NCI Cancer Centers. I've highlighted the SPOREs dedicated to the deadliest cancers.

The nearest NCI center to where you live may not be where you ultimately seek treatment.

But it's a good starting point... and probably 100% better than your neighborhood doctor, hospital, or for-profit cancer center.

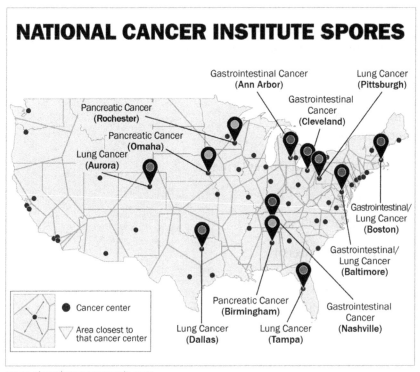

The SPOREs for pancreatic cancer are:

Mayo Clinic
Rochester, Minnesota
(507) 284-2511
www.mayoclinic.org/patient-visitor-guide/minnesota

University of Alabama at Birmingham
Birmingham, Alabama
(800) UAB-0933
www3.ccc.uab.edu/

University of Nebraska Medical Center
Omaha, Nebraska
(402) 559-4000
www.unmc.edu/

The SPOREs for gastrointestinal cancers (including liver, esophagus, and stomach cancer) are:

Case Western Reserve University
Cleveland, Ohio
(216) 844-8797
cancer.case.edu/

Dana-Farber Harvard Cancer Center
Boston, Massachusetts
(877) 420-3951
www.dfhcc.harvard.edu/

Johns Hopkins University
Baltimore, Maryland
(410) 955-5000
www.hopkinsmedicine.org/kimmel_cancer_center/

University of Michigan
Ann Arbor, Michigan
(734) 647-8902
www.mcancer.org/gastrointestinal-cancer/gastrointestinal-cancer-clinic

Vanderbilt University
Nashville, Tennessee
(877) 936-8422
www.vicc.org/

The SPOREs for lung cancer are:

Dana-Farber Harvard Cancer Center
Boston, Massachusetts
(877) 420-3951
www.dfhcc.harvard.edu/

H. Lee Moffitt Cancer Center and Research Institute
Tampa, Florida
(888) 663-3488
moffitt.org/

Johns Hopkins University
Baltimore, Maryland
(410) 955-5000
www.hopkinsmedicine.org/kimmel_cancer_center/

University of Colorado Cancer Center
Aurora, Colorado
(303) 724-3155
www.ucdenver.edu/academics/colleges/medicalschool/centers/
cancercenter/Pages/CancerCenter.aspx

University of Pittsburgh
Pittsburgh, Pennsylvania
(412) 647-2811
www.upci.upmc.edu/

University of Texas/Southwestern Medical Center
Dallas, Texas
(214) 648-3111
www.utsouthwestern.edu/

You can also utilize information from cancer foundations. The Leukemia & Lymphoma Society, for example, has links to hospitals at the forefront of blood-cancer research, information on financial and emotional support, and in-depth information about the different types of blood cancers.

When you're looking for the best place for your treatment, make sure you're looking for places nearby doing clinical trials. Many of the most impressive results... the clues to turning on the Living Cure... have come from these cutting-edge trials...

The Importance of Clinical Trials

Several years ago, researchers from the Dana-Farber Cancer Institute began an international follow-up on advanced melanoma patients who had been treated with a new drug called ipilimumab.

Ipilimumab is a new type of cancer drug that triggers your immune system to fight cancer cells. Think of it like how antibiotics work to fight an infection.

It was the largest and longest-term study of its kind. The lead researcher, Professor Stephen Hodi, said, "Our findings demonstrate that there is a plateau in overall survival, which begins around the third year and extends through to the tenth year."

The analysis found potentially 25% of patients with Stage 4 melanoma can survive up to 10 years when treated with ipilimumab versus the average survival rate of 10%-15%. This is a promising sign for the future of treating other types of cancer using what are known as "monoclonal antibodies." That's why clinical trials, and patients' willingness to partake, are leading the way for the future of cancer treatments.

Some people avoid clinical trials thinking they're expensive or dangerous. Others think clinical trials are meant solely for people who are in advanced stages or haven't responded to standard treatments.

Clinical trials are used to test the effects of cancer treatments on patients.

There are four phases of clinical trials...

Phase I – The drug or treatment is tested to determine dosage, safety, and side effects. This phase is done on healthy people, not those with disease.

Phase II – The drug or treatment is tested for effectiveness and to continue reviewing its safety.

Phase III – The drug or treatment is again tested for effectiveness and side effects and compared with current drugs or treatments.

Phase IV – The drug or treatment is tested for long-term use after it has been licensed and marketed.

Clinical trials are a crucial part of developing new drugs

and treatments. Clinical trials provide benefits for participants as well. They give patients access to new drugs and the best doctors and treatment centers. And – depending on the trials – patients may receive financial compensation.

If you're interested in finding clinical trials, visit ClinicalTrials.gov. The National Institutes of Health maintains this website as a registry and database of trials conducted around the world.

According to the Cancer Research Institute (CRI), only three immunotherapies have been approved to treat cancer. So for most patients, a clinical trial is the only way to try an immunotherapy.

The CRI provides information on cancer immunotherapy clinical trials. You can search the Institute's database of clinical trials here: www.cancerresearch.org/cancer-immunotherapy/clinical-trial-finder. You need an account to access the database. Setting one up is simple. Select a username and password, and provide your e-mail address and two security questions. Then you can start searching for clinical trials. You can also call 1-855-216-0127 to speak with a Clinical Trial Navigator (available Monday through Friday from 8:30 a.m. to 6 p.m. Eastern Time).

Interested in Immunotherapy Clinical Trials?

There are active immunotherapy clinical trials across the country. In fall 2014, both Wake Forest Baptist Health and the University of Tennessee Medical Center are recruiting participants for a study for the effects of immunotherapy on patients with Stage 4 melanoma. These are just two examples out of the many trials.

If you're interested in these trials, contact:

Wake Forest Baptist Health
Stacey Lewis, RN
(336) 713-6927
stalewis@wakehealth.edu

University of Tennessee Medical Center
Shanna Overbey
(865) 305-5281
soverbey@utmck.edu

CRI has also gathered information on current treatments and the impact of immunotherapy on certain cancers. You can see that list here: www.cancerresearch.org/cancer-immunotherapy/impacting-all-cancers.

You can also find clinical trials through major cancer centers like the Dana-Farber Cancer Institute, the Memorial Sloan Kettering Cancer Center, and the MD Anderson Cancer Center.

You can find more about their clinical trials here:

Dana-Farber Cancer Institute
(866) 408-3324
www.dana-farber.org/Research/About-Clinical-Trials.aspx

Memorial Sloan Kettering Cancer Center
(212) 639-2000
www.mskcc.org/cancer-care/clinical-trials

MD Anderson Cancer Center
(877) 632-6789
www.mdanderson.org/patient-and-cancer-information/cancer-information/clinical-trials/clinical-trials-at-md-anderson/index.html

One of the leaders in immunotherapy – Dr. Steve Rosenberg – is involved in several immunotherapy studies at the National Institutes of Health Clinical Center in Bethesda, Maryland, which you can see here: https://ccr.cancer.gov/steven-a-rosenberg?qt-staff_profile_tabs=1.

Clinical trials do, of course, come with some risks you should consider...

The drugs could trigger unexpected side effects, as we explained earlier. Also, your health insurance may not cover the trial, or the drugs may not work for you. But more often than not, the drug costs are included in the trial, and your odds are better than current therapies.

— Chapter 7 —

How to Get Into a Clinical Trial

Once you've decided to join a critical trial, you need to see if you meet the criteria.

There are two types of participants in a trial – healthy volunteers and patient volunteers (though not every trial uses both).

Healthy volunteers have no significant health problems and are used as controls in clinical trials.

Patient volunteers suffer from whatever health issue (like cancer) is being researched and tested in the trial. For example, a trial testing the effects of an immunotherapy drug on breast cancer would need patient volunteers that have breast cancer.

Each trial has "Inclusion/Exclusion" criteria. This information is provided when you find the trial on any of the sites we mentioned above. This criteria is detailed, and you may need the help of your doctor to figure out if you're eligible.

Let's take a look at some of the criteria for the melanoma study we mentioned earlier...

The inclusion criteria (what you need to be a participant) include:

- Histological diagnosis of melanoma. AJCC Stage 4 (any T, any N, M1), metastatic, progressive, refractory, melanoma.

- Serum albumin ≥3.0 gm/dL.

- Patients must be ≥4 weeks since major surgery, radiotherapy, chemotherapy (six weeks if they were treated with nitrosureas) or biotherapy/targeted therapies.

Three Things You Need to Do After a Cancer Diagnosis

You need to do three critical things immediately after an initial diagnosis: Confirm the diagnosis, get the pathology results, and do your research.

First, confirm your diagnosis. Go out and get a second, or even third, opinion. Doctors make mistakes like everyone else. Don't put yourself through dangerous treatments – like radiation and chemotherapy – without the certainty you have cancer.

Second, wait for tissue pathology. If you have a "solid cancer," like breast cancer, waiting for the pathology to determine your cancer type is critical before starting treatment. However, this may not apply if you have a blood disorder like acute leukemia, which often requires urgent treatment.

Third, research, research, and research some more. Find out what your treatment options are, which hospitals lead the field in the cancer you have, and how to join potential trials.

The exclusion criteria (factors that would make you ineligible) include:

- Age < 18 years old.

- Patients who have previously undergone splenectomy.

- Patients with known hepatitis or unstable liver disease, and/or positive serologies for Hepatitis B or C and HIV.

Talk to your doctor and contact the people handling the trial. They can help you determine whether or not you're eligible, if any costs are covered, and if the benefits to you outweigh any risks of the trial.

You May Also Like...

I talk in more detail about immunotherapy and other potentially life-saving medical and general health advice in my *Retirement Millionaire* newsletter.

For more information about *Retirement Millionaire*, call **888-261-2693**. Or go straight to our order form by typing this unique, safe, and secure website address into your Internet browser: www.sbry.co/ok5cnn.

— Part II —

**What You Need to Know
After a Cancer Diagnosis**

Chapter 1

10 Must-Ask Questions for Your Doctor

Regardless whether you end up pursuing a Living Cure treatment... any cancer diagnosis requires immediate action to ensure your survival. At that moment, you're probably shocked and scared... And doctors – often unhelpfully – are flooding you with a textbook's worth of information of what the cancer is and how to treat it.

Before you're completely overwhelmed, remember, doctors are sometimes wrong. They're human and make assumptions about what's most probable and likely.

But you're not a statistic, and you need to make sure you're really getting the care you deserve.

I've consulted experts in the field of cancer and spoken with several general doctors as well about the issues...

Here's what you must ask your doctors after a cancer diagnosis...

1. **"What is my specific diagnosis?"** Your doctor should be able to openly and freely tell you what you have. There shouldn't be any hemming and hawing.

If they think it may be one of two or three things, they should tell you. After you've been told what the doctor thinks you have, demand proof.

2. **"Has my diagnosis been confirmed with pathologic tissue?"** This means they'll need to get a biopsy or blood sample to confirm the cancer diagnosis by looking at real cells from your body.

If the answer is yes, ask to have a copy of the signed report from the pathologist. With the report, you can share it with your regular doctor or even take it to a second doctor for a confirming opinion. You'd be surprised how often pathology samples get lost, misplaced, or mislabeled.

Be sure and wait for this pathology report before starting any therapy. There's no sense in risking your health and life because your cancer doctor thinks the results will be positive. Be sure.

If the answer is no, ask why not. If you've been told you have cancer, but your doctor refuses to get tissue to confirm it... get right up and leave. Find a second doctor immediately who will confirm your diagnosis. There are a few exceptions, like pancreatic cancer... But your cancer doctors better have a good reason as to why they won't do a biopsy.

Why Wait for Pathology?

Waiting for a tissue pathology to define your cancer type is critical before starting treatment for almost all "solid" cancers. But a few cancers, mostly blood disorders such as acute leukemia (or Burkitt's lymphoma) are emergencies and require starting treatment immediately.

If your doctor says it's emergent and time to treat, don't mess around. But if your doctor can't tell you definitively that you should be treated immediately, get a biopsy and confirmation from the pathologist before starting the occasionally deadly therapies.

3. **"What is my prognosis?"**
Ask for the five-year survival (FYS) or 10-year life expectancy. This is one of the hardest things to get from most doctors because your doctor is worried that whatever he tells you will be interpreted as a death sentence. For example, if he tells you the FYS was 80%, do you "hear" that number or did you hear you have a 20% chance of dying?

Once you have this number, it can help you consider your treatment options as well as what life changes, if any, you want to make and how quickly you need to make them.

And when you get the number, ask your cancer doctor and regular doctor to explain what the number means. It should become painfully clear that the number is an average and may not even be close to your actual outcome. There are hundreds of stories of people with very low FYS that go into remission and live another 20 years. So don't let the numbers shake you... Just take them for what they are.

4. **"What is the recommended treatment?"** Make sure your doctor explains and spells out (preferably in writing) what he recommends for treatment. And more importantly...

5. **"Is it in the National Cancer Center Network (NCCN) guidelines?"** Millions of dollars and hours go into figuring out what the best and most likely outcomes will be for cancer treatments. The NCCN is a compilation of smart folks that spend tons of time thinking about the pros and cons of different treatment plans.

If you're recommended a non-NCCN plan, be sure there's science to back it up. And ask for proof and background of the reasons for going off the path.

6. **"What are the top three centers in this field of cancer?"** You may not have the resources to go to these centers for treatment – the costs and travel may be outside your budget – but these centers may have the resources to help you. The world is getting smaller, and you may be able to be a part of cutting-edge and important research from these centers while you stay in your hometown.

Clinical trials often pay for medications. These trials usually come from the top centers... Please ask who is doing the cutting-edge work in your cancer field. If your cancer doctor is offended or bored by the idea or effort needed to get you involved, get another doctor – or contact the centers yourself.

7. **"How many people have this disease in the U.S.?"** If it's less than 5,000 people in the U.S., get to a major cancer center right away. If you have a rare and deadly cancer, you'll want the best in the field thinking and working on your cancer.

8. **"How many patients like me have you seen in your career, and how many have you treated successfully?"** This relates to the question above. Whatever your doctor says, get him to put it in writing. Make him be truthful and honest with you about his success.

When I was training, it would drive me crazy to watch doctor after doctor lie about their level of experience and success. Most doctors, even surgeons, don't keep good records of their procedures or treatments. But ask anyway, and see what you get.

If you see squirming and evasiveness... find another doctor who will at least tell you he hasn't kept a perfect track but can offer an approximate level of experience and success.

9. **"Are there clinical trials for my diagnosis?"** It is helpful to know about alternative ideas about treating your cancer. And you may be able to get financial assistance for parts of your cutting-edge treatment. You can read about the possible trials on the government website here: www. nih.gov/health/clinicaltrials/index.htm.

10. **"What's the goal of treatment? Palliative versus cure?"** It's important to know whether you're going to get treatment that will make you comfortable or try to cure you. If it's the former, you'll want to get your affairs in order sooner than later.

As you consider asking your doctor these 10 critical questions, I encourage you to do a few things to make the process easier and clearer for you. These tips will go a long way to help you.

First, it's important that on every visit to your doctor, you do several things...

Have your doctor give you a written diagnosis on a piece of paper.

Always bring a friend or close family member with you. It's so hard to pay attention to everything going on all the time during a visit. And different people hear different things in different ways. A friend there in the room with you for support can remind and encourage you to keep asking the 10 questions. A friend can also help you recall what the doctor said or meant when you're reflecting on it after the visits.

Take written notes at each office visit. Ask for your doctor to write things down for you if they aren't clear. He should be willing to spend time with you and help you get the information you need about your situation.

Finally, it's critical that you consider the issues surrounding death and dying at this point. Please discuss end-of-life issues with your next of kin (and family). This means doing things like executing a living will and health-care power of attorney.

I hope these critical questions and tips will make your path through the issues surrounding a cancer diagnosis a little easier. As you contemplate your mortality and the short time you have on this earth, I also hope these ideas help you communicate more easily with all those around you to face the decisions you'll be making together.

By talking about this stuff openly with your doctor, friends, and family, you'll feel safer and calmer. Find a doctor who'll work honestly with you, and your chances of healing improve.

Chapter 2

Understand Your Risk of Cancer

Risk factors vary from cancer to cancer. Some – like leukemia – aren't strongly linked to genetics. Other cancers have a clear genetic link. About 10% of breast-cancer patients can link the cancer back to abnormal genes they received from their parents.

But we do know risk factors that increase your odds of getting cancer regardless of type. They include:

- Radiation exposure

- Poor diet (one that lacks fruits and vegetables)

- Obesity

- Alcohol consumption above moderate levels

- Smoking/tobacco use

While you can't change your genetics, you can control the risk factors above.

Exposure to radiation comes from numerous sources. One is the sun... The sun gives off electromagnetic waves – you've probably heard of ultraviolet (UV) rays, which are just one type. The UV rays are the electromagnetic waves that cause sunburn.

While some sun in necessary – it's one of the ways our bodies get vitamin D – too much can cause sunburn. Sunburn doubles your risk of developing skin cancers. So while you need to get a little bit of sun, you don't want to overdo it. That's why I recommend avoiding the sun between 10:30 a.m. and 2:30 p.m., when the sun is strongest.

But you should be wary of the amount of radiation you receive from voluntary sources...

While they're useful, x-rays come with a big risk in the form of radiation. Any amount of radiation leads to an increased risk of developing several different cancers. This includes CT scans, mammograms, and the scanners at airports.

And eating healthy is key..

"Cruciferous" vegetables – like broccoli, Brussels sprouts, and cabbage – are packed with beneficial chemicals. They fight inflation and can reduce your risk of cardiovascular disease and diabetes.

Berries are also effective at fighting cancer... Blueberries, strawberries, and raspberries all have incredible health benefits. From improving memory to boosting your immune system to keeping your eyes healthy, berries are an important food to include in your everyday diet.

A poor diet can also lead to obesity, another risk factor. The World Health Organization (WHO) says obesity is the second-most avoidable cause of cancer (behind tobacco). According to Cancer Research UK, obese women are 30% more likely to develop breast cancer than women who have a healthy weight.

A good diet and exercise are key to maintaining a healthy weight.

Avoid foods that are high calorie and low nutritional value like sugar, white bread, and white rice. I call these foods "white killers."

When you eat these so-called "high glycemic index" foods, your body signals the pancreas to produce extra insulin. Insulin also results in fat production.

The insulin secreted into the blood stream triggers a host of things – a decrease of magnesium and an increase of sodium in the blood. Insulin also increases inflammatory molecules in the blood.

White sugar is a food I avoid eating at all costs. While it is a carbohydrate – the fuel that runs our bodies – it contains no vitamins and minerals. (And I'd rather get my carbs from a healthier source like whole grains or fruit.)

The other two killers, white rice and white bread, are both carbohydrates that have been stripped of their natural health benefits.

White rice is simply brown rice stripped of the outer layers (husk, bran, and germ). These parts contain most of the benefits of rice... like the fiber. The rice is then bleached to enhance the white color.

White bread is loaded with calories and sugar. It offers little nutritional benefit because it lacks whole grains. And like rice, it's full of chemicals that make it look pristine and appetizing.

I'll eat brown and wild rice and whole-grain breads or nothing at all. Some of my favorite breads have 12 grains or more and look (and feel) like fiberboard from the lumber mill. If you don't like the texture or taste of fully whole-grain bread, look for some with three or more grains. (They have a softer, less grainy texture than my favorites, but still have benefits.)

In moderation, alcohol is good for you. Among other things, drinks like beer and wine raise high-density lipoprotein (HDL), or "good" cholesterol, that is believed to aid heart health.

Moderate alcohol intake also decreases the risk of dementia by 23%. Having a drink or two, three to four times per week also lowers the risk of blood clotting. A 2009 study even found moderate drinking cuts the risk of developing gallstones by a third.

But don't drink much more than that... Overconsumption of alcohol can lead to anemia, and it increases the risk of cancer (like liver or mouth cancer), cardiovascular disease, and cirrhosis.

And smoking is associated with cancer of the lung, kidney, bladder, mouth, and more. The best advice is to never start smoking. But if you're already a smoker and you want to quit, visit smokefree.gov to learn how.

Final Thoughts

I truly believe the latest developments in immunotherapy will not only give us powerful tools in fighting cancer... but will ultimately take the terror and fatality out of cancer diagnoses.

I'm confident the information I've given you in this booklet could change the lives of many people facing cancer diagnosis.

I hope you have found this information to be as valuable as I believe it is...

If so, you may be interested in related research we've done into the opportunities in investing in companies driving advances in the Living Cure.

For example, one large pharmaceutical company is leading the way in immunotherapy. This company has put all its chips on the Living Cure – selling off other parts of the business to direct more research and acquisition dollars to this breakthrough trend. And *it owns the first – and by far, the largest – commercially available immunotherapy drug, with sales expected to reach $2 billion a year by 2018.*

It's a low-risk way to capture some solid financial gains as the immunotherapy tidal wave hits the market.

I profiled this company in an exclusive report for my *Retirement Millionaire* subscribers titled: "Killing Cancer: How to Invest in the Most Important Medical Megatrend of the 21st Century."

In addition, a small number of companies are going to control the technologies that turn cancer from a killer into a chronic aliment... and then possibly make some cancers a thing of the past. Investing in the right companies today could result in triple-digit returns as their work develops...

Retirement Millionaire subscribers also have access to a special report detailing the top four small stocks to invest in this trend.

If you'd like to learn more about subscribing to *Retirement Millionaire* – and how to access these other immunotherapy reports – you can call Stansberry Research's knowledgeable Member Services team at **888-261-2693**. Or you can subscribe online here:/www.sbry.co/ok5cnn..

You won't have to watch any video or presentation.

Appendix:
Published Studies and
Related Research

Abramson Cancer Center of the University of Pennsylvania. (n.d.). *T-Cell immunotherapy for leukemia*. Retrieved October 15, 2014, from http://www.penncancer.org/tcelltherapy/

Ackerman, T. (2014, April 16). Jim Allison confronts cancer, critics with immunotherapy. *SFGate*. Retrieved October 15, 2014, from http://www.sfgate.com/health/article/Jim-Allison-confronts-cancer-critics-with-5405290.php

Agence France-Presse. (2014, June 2). New immunotherapy treatments show dramatic progress in fight against cervical cancer. *Raw Story*. Retrieved October 16, 2014, from http://www.rawstory.com/rs/2014/06/new-immunotherapy-treatments-show-dramatic-progress-in-fight-against-cervical-cancer/

American Cancer Society. (2014, September 5). Types of cancer immunotherapy. *American Cancer Society*. Retrieved October 14, 2014, from http://www.cancer.org/treatment/treatmentsandsideeffects/treatmenttypes/immunotherapy/immunotherapy-types

American Cancer Society. (2014, September 5). Cancer immunotherapy. *American Cancer Society*. Retrieved October 14, 2014, from http://www.cancer.org/acs/groups/cid/documents/webcontent/003013-pdf.pdf

American Cancer Society. (2014, May 13). What are the different types of cancer treatment? *American Cancer Society*. Retrieved October 14, 2014, from http://www.cancer.org/treatment/understandingyourdiagnosis/talkingaboutcancer/whensomeoneyouknowhascancer/when-somebody-you-know-has-cancer-cancer-treatment-questions

Baum, A., Dainty, M., Jerman, J., et al. (2013, May 23). Immunotherapy – the beginning of the end for cancer. Citi Research. Retrieved October 15, 2014, from https://www.citivelocity.com/citigps/OpArticleDetail.action?recordId=209

Cambridge Healthtech Institute's Inaugural Combination Cancer Immunotherapy Conference. August 12-13, 2014. (2014, August 12). *The Ninth Annual Immunotherapies and Vaccine Summit.* Retrieved October 15, 2014, from http://www.imvacs.com/Combination-Cancer-Immunotherapy/

Cancer causes and risk factors. (n.d.). *National Cancer Institute.* Retrieved October 14, 2014, from http://www.cancer.gov/cancertopics/causes

Clinical trial finder. (2014). *Cancer Research Institute.* Retrieved October 15, 2014, from http://www.cancerresearch.org/cancer-immunotherapy/clinical-trial-finder

"Doctor, can we talk?": tips for communicating with your health care team (n.d.). *CancerCare.* Retrieved October 15, 2014, from http://www.cancercare.org/publications/53-doctor_can_we_talk_tips_for_communicating_with_your_health_care_team

Fellner, C. (2012). Ipilimumab (Yervoy) Prolongs Survival In Advanced Melanoma. *Pharmacy and Therapeutics, 37*(9), 503-511, 530. Retrieved October 16, 2014, from http://www.ncbi.nlm.nih.gov/pmc/articles/PMC3462607/#b16-ptj3709503

Grady, D. (2012, December 9). In Girl's Last Hope, Altered Immune Cells Beat Leukemia. *The New York Times.* Retrieved October 16, 2014, from http://www.nytimes.com/2012/12/10/health/a-breakthrough-against-leukemia-using-altered-t-cells.html?_r=0

Groopman, J. (2012, April 23). The T-Cell army. *The New Yorker.* Retrieved October 15, 2014, from http://www.newyorker.com/magazine/2012/04/23/the-t-cell-army

Herper, M. (2013, May 15). With 'cell death' drugs, Bristol-Myers may win no matter what. *Forbes.* Retrieved October 15, 2014, from http://www.forbes.com/sites/matthewherper/2013/05/15/experimental-cell-death-cancer-drugs-generate-excitement/

Hoption Cann, S. A., van Netten, J. P., & van Netten, C. (2003). Dr. William Coley and tumor regression: a place in history or in the future. *Postgraduate Medical Journal, 79,* 672-680.

Hosemann, S. (2011, January 1). Compass: Metastatic Melanoma. *OncoLog*. Retrieved October 16, 2014, from http://www2.mdanderson.org/depts/oncolog/articles/11/1-jan/1-11-compass.html

Kalos, M., & June, C. (2013). Adoptive T cell transfer for cancer immunotherapy in the era of synthetic biology. *Immunity*, 39(1), 49-60. Retrieved October 14, 2014, from http://dx.doi.org/10.1016/j.immuni.2013.07.002

Ledford, H. (2014). Cancer treatment: The killer within. *Nature*, 508(7494), 24-26.

Marchione, M. (2013, December 7). Gene therapy scores big wins against blood cancers. *Yahoo! News*. Retrieved October 16, 2014, from https://news.yahoo.com/gene-therapy-scores-big-wins-against-blood-cancers-160100028.html

Marchione, M. (2014, June 2). Doctors use immune therapy against cervical cancer. *The Big Story*. Retrieved October 16, 2014, from http://bigstory.ap.org/article/doctors-use-immune-therapy-against-cervical-cancer

Mary Elizabeth Williams: Conquering Cancer with the Immune System. (n.d.). *Cancer Research Institute*. Retrieved October 16, 2014, from http://cancerresearch.org/news-publications/video-gallery/mary-elizabeth-williams-conquering-cancer-with-th

McCoy, K. D., & Gros, G. L. (1999). The role of CTLA-4 in the regulation of T cell immune responses. *Immunology and Cell Biology*, 77(1), 1-10. Retrieved October 14, 2014, from http://dx.doi.org/10.1046/j.1440-1711.1999.00795.x

NCI's Dr. Steven Rosenberg talks TILs in breast cancer and much more. (2014, September 15). *The Oncology Report*. Retrieved October 15, 2014, from http://www.oncologypractice.com/the-oncology-report/home/article/video-ncis-dr-steven-rosenberg-talks-tils-in-breast-cancer-and-much-more/bafa7a5c134f48dde4151deb8ac1e1e9.html

National Comprehensive Cancer Network. (n.d.). Understanding your risk of developing secondary cancers. Retrieved October 15, 2014, from http://www.nccn.org/patients/resources/life_after_cancer/understanding.aspx

Relapsed Leukemia: Emily's Story. (n.d.). *The Children's Hospital of Philadelphia*. Retrieved October 16, 2014, from http://www.chop.edu/stories/relapsed-leukemia-emilys-story#.VD-4JhaK1YU

U.S. Food and Drug Administration. (2014, September 4). FDA approves Keytruda for advanced melanoma. *FDA Press Releases*. Retrieved October 14, 2014, from http://www.fda.gov/NewsEvents/Newsroom/PressAnnouncements/ucm412802.htm

Whitehead, E. (2014, May 10). Two Years Cancer Free! *Emily Emma Whitehead: My Journey Fighting Leukemia Two Years Cancer Free*. Retrieved October 16, 2014, from http://emilywhitehead.com/2014/05/two-years-cancer-free/

Williams, M. E. (n.d.). Hilarious Misadventures at Stage 4 – And Beyond. *Mary Elizabeth Williams*. Retrieved October 16, 2014, from http://www.maryelizabethwilliams.net/8201.html

More From Dr. Eifrig

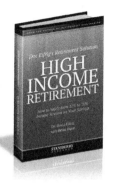

High Income Retirement: How to Safely Earn 12% to 20% Income Streams on Your Savings

For the first time ever, Dr. Eifrig reveals his proven options strategy in one easy-to-read manual. This book gives the step-by-step details of the investing strategy he used to close 136 consecutive winning positions... a track record of profitable trading recommendations unmatched in the financial publishing industry.

High Income Retirement contains everything you need to know to begin using this strategy. Doc outlines how stock options work and how to use them to reduce risk. He also debunks the most common misperceptions of stock options and explains why most people misuse them. Finally, he walks readers through exactly how to make his safe, profitable trades.

If you want to trade like the professionals, this book is a must-read.

To order your own copy, call **888-261-2693** and use **reference code BOOKS100**.

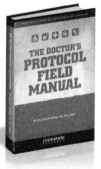

The Doctor's Protocol Field Manual

The Doctor's Protocol Field Manual is one of the most valuable books in America today... packed with dozens of secrets, ideas, and strategies that can save you and your family in a time of crisis.

You won't hear these easy ways to guard against threats to your wellbeing from the media... because an entire industry has emerged to encourage dread and pray on these fears. So Dr. Eifrig constructed a scientific protocol for surviving just about any crisis that may befall you...

In the manual, you'll learn surprisingly simple strategies and tactics for survival, like...

- Four antibiotics you must have in your home.
- What to do if someone starts shooting in a public place.
- The most important thing to do when a loved one is injured.
- How to legally hide money and assets from the government.

Dr. Eifrig moves beyond hype and fear to real, actionable steps for survival and prosperity in the midst of any crisis.

To order your own copy, call **888-261-2693** and use **reference code BOOKS100**.

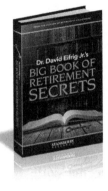

Dr. David Eifrig Jr.'s
Big Book of Retirement Secrets

It's time to look at retirement in a completely different way.

Erase the dangerous information you've been spoon-fed since you were too young to know the difference about your money, your health, and how things work in America.

Dangerous beliefs like, *"Go to a good school and get a job with a big corporation, and it takes care of your retirement"*... *"Buy mutual funds and everything will be fine by the time you retire"*... or *"Wall Street will take care of your money"*...

Here's the truth: The only one who will take care of you in your retirement is you.

That's why Dr. David "Doc" Eifrig Jr. wrote the *Big Book of Retirement Secrets*. It's a treasure trove of wisdom and well-researched ideas for living a life full of health, freedom, and abundance...

In it, Dr. Eifrig takes an in-depth look at six loopholes that will help you save and even earn money in your retirement. He also analyzes several investment strategies and health tips and secrets that will help you live a happy, healthy, and wealthy life.

To order your own copy, call **888-261-2693** and use **reference code BOOKS100**.

How to Follow Dr. Eifrig's Latest Research and Ideas

Dr. Eifrig writes three newsletters for Stansberry Research: *Retirement Millionaire, Retirement Trader,* and *Income Intelligence.* These are some of the best and most popular advisories in America...

- Doc gives more than investment advice in **Retirement Millionaire**. He shows subscribers how to invest and collect "free cash" without ever worrying about money again. But each month, he also gives invaluable tips for travel, health, and living a happy life.

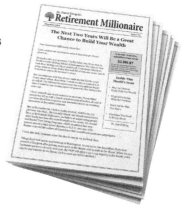

For example, Doc has shown *Retirement Millionaire* subscribers how to collect "rent" from investments... two foods that prevent cancer... how to receive a free wine vacation... a simple secret to save up to 90% on local attractions... how to get free golf... and much more.

If you want to know more ways to live a wealthier, healthier retirement, try a risk-free trial subscription to *Retirement Millionaire* for just $39, **call 888-261-2693**

Or you can go directly to our *Retirement Millionaire* order form by typing this unique, safe, and secure website address into your Internet browser: www.sbry.co/ok5cnn.

- In ***Retirement Trader***, Dr. Eifrig teaches subscribers a trading secret that can produce quick gains in a matter of minutes. It's one of the safest – yet misunderstood – strategies in the markets. Yet 99% of investors have never heard about it.

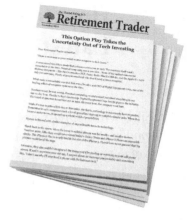

Doc used this strategy to close 136 consecutive winning positions for his subscribers... a track record unparalleled in the financial newsletter industry. Once you see how simple this strategy is, you'll never look at trading the same way again.

Retirement Trader is Dr. Eifrig's most elite service, selling for $3,000 per year. To join this exclusive advisory and learn how to trade like the professionals... **call 888-261-2693**.

- ***Income Intelligence*** has a
  simple goal: Help readers find the
  safest, most profitable ways to
  earn income on their savings. It's
  a full-service approach to income
  investing that covers dividend
  stocks, municipal bonds, MLPs,
  REITs, and other alternative
  investments.

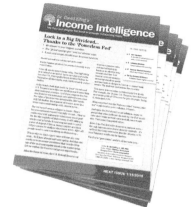

Dr. Eifrig uses several proprietary
indicators, which help him spot
little-known investments that can achieve near double-digit
returns with unbelievably low risk.

This service is designed for investors of every level, with simple
explanations and investments that are easy to make in any
brokerage account.

If you want the opportunity to earn high yields on safe
investments and understand all the financial forces affecting your
income, try a risk-free trial subscription to *Income Intelligence*
for $149, **call 888-261-2693**.

Or you can go directly to our *Income Intelligence* order form by
typing this unique, safe, and secure website address into your
Internet browser: www.sbry.co/dQl7XC.

More from Stansberry Research

The World's Greatest Investment Ideas

The Stansberry Research Trader's Manual

World Dominating Dividend Growers:
Income Streams That Never Go Down

Secrets of the Natural Resource Market:
How to Set Yourself up for Huge Returns in
Mining, Energy, and Agriculture

The Stansberry Research Guide to Investment Basics

The Stansberry Research Starter's Guide for New Investors